# *ALZHEIMER'S, SCIENCE AND GOD*

Rev. H. Kroeger
Chapel of Miracles

© Rev. Hanna Kroeger, 1990

ISBN 1-883713-10-2

# Alzheimer's Disease

Alzheimer's Disease, a progressive, degenerative disease, attacks the brain resulting in impaired memory, thinking and behavior. Over four million American adults are now affected.

According to Alzheimer's Association President, Edward Truschke, "Families of Alzheimer patients face tremendous emotional, physical and financial hardships. As the disease progresses, the task of providing 'round the clock care can be overwhelming, especially for those who bear the burden alone."

# Facing the Facts

- Approximately 10 percent of people 65 and over have "probable" Alzheimer's; 47 percent of those over 85 have the disease.

- $123.4 million in federal funds was allocated to Alzheimer's research in 1989, compared with $5.1 million allocated in 1978.

- An estimated 10 to 30 percent of Alzheimer's patients have the type that is inherited.

- Stress from looking after Alzheimer's patients makes caregivers more vulnerable to infectious disease.

# Stages of Alzheimer's Disease

**First Stage:** The disease begins very gradually, with minor symptoms and mood changes. Often no one notices anything wrong.

Patient seems to have less energy, less drive, less spontaneity; is slower to learn, slower to react, forgets some words. Patient loses temper easily, with little cause. Seeks the familiar, avoids the new.

**Second Stage:** The patient can still perform familiar activities, but may need help with complicated tasks.

Speech and understanding are much slower. Patient finds it very hard to make decisions; may lose the thread of a story. He or She becomes insensitive to feelings of others and avoids situations that may lead to failure.

**Third Stage:** The patient is now obviously disabled. Memory of distant past may still be very clear, but memory of recent past is very poor. Patient forgets where he is, forgets date, time, season. Instructions must be very clear, repeated often. Patient invents words, doesn't recognize familiar people.

**Fourth Stage:** The patient needs help with all activities. Memory is very poor. Patient cannot find his way around at all. Does not recognize people, even family members and close friends. May lose control of bowels and bladder.

# *Forgetfulness:*
## *Not Necessarily an*
## *Early Sign of Alzheimer's*

First, the good news: If forgetfulness is beginning to bother you or a
loved one, it probably is not caused by Alzheimer's. The reason:
Realizing that you've forgotten something is a fairly reliable sign that
your mental faculties are simply aging normally.

In contrast, the Alzheimer's patient is usually aware that *something*
is wrong—but doesn't know what it might be. Forgetful people tend
to call attention to their lapses by deploring them or joking about
them; the Alzheimer's patient is much more likely to behave as if
everything is alright.

The first noticeable sign of Alzheimer's is much more likely to be
uncharacteristic changes in mood. The patient may be unusually
irritable and angry, or perhaps confused and quiet.

Memory loss is a gradual slowing down of brain function which
occurs normally with age, causing older people to need more time to
learn a new fact or remember an old one.

In contrast, the Alzheimer's patient slowly, but progressively, loses
all mental function, so that the person who once did something well,
now does it badly—or not at all. This loss of skills, along with the
unusual mood swings, eventually becomes too obvious to ignore. At
this point, the family realizes that something must be wrong and it's
time to see a doctor.

# Three Out of Ten Cases Are Misdiagnosed: Why?

Why do doctors misdiagnose an alarming 30% of all Alzheimer's patients? The answer is simple: Alzheimer's is very difficult to diagnose correctly:

Alzheimer's lacks a "biological marker." Whereas tuberculosis produces a bacteria that can be studied under a microscope and high pressure within the eyes is a reliable sign of glaucoma, there is no easily identifiable biological change which signals the onset of Alzheimer's. Instead, the doctor must be a medical detective.

A good doctor will test for every known condition that might cause confusion and memory loss. Once those are ruled out, the only possibility left is Alzheimer's. This is called "diagnosis by exclusion."

**Depression** can be mistaken for Alzheimer's disease. Not all depressed patients are obviously "sad." Some express depression by seeming slow to understand and acting confused. Depression is a common—and completely normal—response to certain traumatic events, such as the death of a spouse or loved one, or loss of a job. Antidepressant drugs and professional counseling can often renew one's enjoyment of life.

**Endocrine and metabolic disorders** can spark symptoms which closely resemble those of Alzheimer's. One common—and readily treatable—example is hyperthyroidism.

**Alcoholism, malnutrition and vitamin deficiencies** can cause confusion and forgetfulness. Abstaining from alcohol and establishing a wholesome diet may bring about a complete recovery.

**Many illnesses** can cause confusion and diminished mental capacity. Examples: Appendicitis, infections, the flu, heart attack (in fact, confusion may be the *only* sign of heart attack in an elderly person; some 15% experience no chest pain).

**Toxic substances in the environment** may cause dementia. A change in use of pesticides or other chemicals should be included in any case history concerning a confused person.

**A brain tumor or blood clot** can cause confused behavior. Even a minor head injury that went unnoticed could be the underlying cause of dementia.

**A series of small strokes** can cause what is called "multi-infarct dementia" ("infarct" is the name for a small area of tissue which dies because of loss of blood supply). At the time of the stroke itself, the patient may have no symptoms other than a few moments of faintness or dizziness. Thereafter, the lack of blood to certain portions of the brain produces a loss of ability which develops a pattern—perhaps sudden and definite at first, followed by some improvement, followed by another pronounced loss. A patient may lose only one particular skill while all others remain intact. (There's no cure, but the underlying risk factors can be controlled by lowering blood pressure, a healthy diet, and getting regular exercise. In some cases, diminished or lost abilities can be improved with physical therapy.)

**Many incurable neurological disorders**—Huntington's disease, Pick's disease, Parkinson's disease, multiple sclerosis—may be mistaken for Alzheimer's. That is why an accurate diagnosis is so important. Ask your physician for help.

# *After the Diagnosis: Now What?*

A diagnosis of Alzheimer's is a shock to everyone. It's important to recognize that you, the patient, and all other family members will need time simply to absorb the news.

A caring doctor will tell you about helpful resources in your community at the time of diagnosis. But, since you may be too upset to understand what he's saying, it's a good idea to schedule a follow-up visit in a couple of weeks—either with the doctor or with a specially trained social worker.

You may also want to gather the family together now, so everyone can have a chance to express their reactions to the news and discuss how they think they can best help. You may be able to cope without much assistance in the beginning, but it's important to let family members know help is both needed and wanted.

# Alzheimer's and Science

There is no medicine known that could and would heal Alzheimer's. There is no procedure, operation or such known to eliminate Alzheimer's disease, therefore we have to look at the latest research on Alzheimer's disease. I am reporting the work of several researchers. Dr. Daniel Perl, Neuropathologist of New York, reports that this disease is not simple.

Dr Perl says that the brain contains billions of nerve cells, or neurons, which communicate among themselves chemically via branch-like outgrowths called axons and dendrites. Normal brain function requires that various neuron groups produce particular chemical transmitters, and that the transmitters pass freely between cells at the "synapses" where their branches meet.

Alzheimer's is a breakdown of the system that produces the neurotransmitter acetylcholine. Autopsies of victims' brains show shortages of the enzyme that prompts cells to make this crucial messenger—some brains contain as little as 10 percent of the normal amount—and the degree of deficiency corresponds directly to the degree of dementia.

Other investigators suspect that Alzheimer's is triggered by some environmental toxin. The reason aluminum gets so much attention is that abnormal accumulations of the metal are often found inside the same neurons as the telltale tangles.

Perl, of New York's Mt. Sinai Medical Center, clearly identified aluminum deposits in Alzheimer's brains in 1980. He has since linked such deposits to two other brain diseases (amyotrophic lateral sclerosis and parkinsonism-dementia) that are prevalent in aluminum-rich regions of the Western Pacific.

Despite these tantalizing links, few of Perl's colleagues share his enthusiasm for the aluminum hypothesis. Exposure can't be the key to Alzheimer's, they say, for aluminum is the most abundant metal in the earth's crust. We all ingest it constantly in our food and water, but our intestinal systems protect us by refusing to digest it. Perl readily acknowledges as much (and that's why he doesn't worry about aluminum cookware). He warns, however, that aluminum comes in many forms, some of which may infiltrate the nervous system by way of the nose.

In an experiment designed to test that idea, Perl stuffed sponges soaked with aluminum lactate into rabbits' nasal passages. After four weeks, he killed the rabbits and found that aluminum had, in fact, accumulated in their neural tissue. He is now looking for evidence that humans absorb the metal by some similar mechanism. "We know very little about what we're exposed to in the way of airborne aluminum," he says, "so there are many question marks here."

# These are scientific facts on Aluminum:

## ALUMINUM POISON

Concerned health practicioners in the U.S.A. and Canada are urging their patrons to avoid aluminum containing products. Why?

Aluminum has a predisposition to affect neuronal tissue. Many tests done on animals showed that behavior and memory in test animals suffered as the aluminum level was increased in the lymph and the brain.

Many researchers feel that aluminum is the major culprit in Alzheimers Disease, a disease of dementia, forgetfulness and senility.

Autopsies showed that Alzheimers Disease afflicted individuals had accumulated 6 times as much aluminum in the brain as healthy people.

I urge you not to take a chance. Throw away your aluminum pots, your beer and soft drinks in aluminum containers. Dr. Berlyne, Den Ari and others stated: "The practice of cooking in aluminum utensils and wrapping foods in aluminum foil may result in gross changes in the aluminum content of food before ingestion."

**Aluminum is also found in:**

Antiacids

Baking powder

Toothpaste

Antiperspirants

Also, numerous cities add aluminum salt to drinking water to reduce the cloudiness of it. It makes the water cosmetically pleasing.

**Other Symptoms of aluminum poison may include:**

a) Dryness of mouth

b) Stomach pain

c) Stomach ulcers

d) Hard Stool and/or with small hardened pieces, "feces stones"

e) Pain in spleen area

f) Children cry a lot

g) Kidney problem, especially the right kidney

**What to do about aluminum poison.**

Antidote No. I:

Homeopathic Aluminae

6X        30X

Antidote No. II:

*Herb Formula:*
Pumpkin Seeds
Okra
Rhubarb root
Cayenne pepper
Peppermint
Dulse
Tradename: METALINE

Antidote No. III:

    Co Enzyme International

These are co-enzyme minerals in an aqueous extraction of naturally chelated colloidal minerals. These minerals are derived from an ancient sea bed mineral deposit. The action of colloidal aluminum with other enzymes removes aluminum deposits on the order of God's law, "Like attracts like."

Many illnesses, including tumors good or bad, are at the end of aluminum accumulations. By removing and transmuting aluminum, the body can rid itself from all kinds of troubles. This is the teaching of Dr. John Ray.


## ARSENIC POISONING

### Another factor was found:

Arsenic poisoning: many household and garden pesticides contain arsenoxide.

Acute arsenic poison has to be treated at once in the emergency room and is not discussed here. However, chronic arsenic poison is rarely discovered, and hardly ever mentioned:

Here are the chronic arsenic poison symptoms:

1. Sweetish metallic taste

2. Garlicky odor to breath and stool

3. Constriction of throat

4. Difficulties in swallowing

5. Burning pains in esophagus, stomach, and sometimes bowel

6. Muscle spasms

7. Pain in muscles of back

The spine is pulled out of line so that people have to go for adjustments over and over again. ("Adjustments do not hold.") Elkium and Faky said arsenic, the element arsenic, is an active enzyme inhibiter.*

Symptoms of chronic arsenic poisoning are also:

1. Mild gastrointestinal disturbances

2. Anorexia

3. Low grade fever (changes in white blood count)

4. Weakness

5. Catarrhal symptoms (nose, throat, eyes)

6. Brittle nails

7. Loss of hair

8. Localized edema (eyelids) of the liver

9. Nervousness

Since arsenic has a constricting effect on the muscle structure, and loves to lodge in muscles, the most outstanding symptom is the constant backache.

**ARSENIC ALSO SETTLES IN THE BRAIN DISLODGING THE PHOSPHORUS WHICH IS NEEDED FOR PROPER BRAIN FUNCTIONING.**

*See my book entitled "God Helps Those That Help Themselves."

# *What To Do*

Arsenic: If you can find Mexican raw sugar, take 1 tsp. 3x daily.
Arsenicum 3x to 30x does the job. The herb combination *Metaline*
transmutes almost all metals.

Very helpful is the tea from South Africa called Harpagophytum.
This tea washes out metallic poisons as well as chemical poisons. It
carries the rare combination of 3 active ingredients: Flukoside,
Fruran, and Pyror.

There is an old time natural remedy used over centuries and
centuries: Healing Earth, Bentonite, Luvas, and Bolus-alba.

# *Alzheimers and God*

All Alzheimer's patients suffer from arterial blockage. Arteries leading to the brain and also inside the brain are blocked: in short, ateriosclerosis. Since this cannot be operated on, natural means have to be employed. I prefer "Circu-Flow" to everything else, which is a God-given formula, a blessing to mankind.

## What is Circu-Flow?

God in His Mercy reached down to us mortals to heal us and free us from our ailments.

In my life I learned that everything Our Lord does, works. So, the Herbal Chelation (which I never claimed was my formula) works. It is Our Lord's formula.

It was in the rush hour of the day when a man approached me asking how he could avoid a bypass operation. "I have four children," he said. "I am not insured. Is there anything I could do to open the arteries?"

I had read an excerpt from a French medical journal in which the benefit of Equisitum (horsetail) was described. It stated Equisitum just ground up should not be taken as it is, but by boiling it takes on a different healing property for the arteries.

I had purchased the French product and I had tried it on myself and my husband, but it had done nothing spectacular, so I had put it aside. So, when this man approached me for help, I had to say "No, I have nothing to offer." He looked at me with deep eyes, desperate for help. He had reached out and I said, "No, I have nothing for you." He dropped his head and so did I. "Jesus, help," I murmured and here the heavens opened. "Take Equisitum concentrate, Hawthorn, Aloe Vera gel." I listened and that was Our Lord's instruction.

I ran after the man who was already half a block down the road. I caught up with him. Breathlessly, I told him to return. Our Lord had given the formula for him.

His eyes expressed doubt. Reluctantly he returned and I filled his bag with the items I was instructed to give.

Ten days later he returned. "I feel so much better," he said. "I want to pay for the items you gave me." Another three weeks and he was free of his troubles.

# *There is God!*

The candles flickered in the Holy Shrine at the Chapel of Miracles. It was early dawn, no one up, no sound, not even the early morning wind had come up. I asked our Lord for help in Alzheimer's disease. I knew that cryptomycosis was the missing link. I had worked diligently to find an herb or a combination of herbs for cryptomycosis, but all my efforts were in vain. And then our Lord sent help! This is when I grasped that Crypto was a spindel cell fungus. I also found it to be present in other diseases, such as AIDS and some types of cancer. I was instructed to take consecrated distilled water, and add a few drops of alcohol and invoke a number which was given in vision before my very eyes, "shake well and give 15 drops, 3 times daily." The candle flickered, the morning wind had become active, a rooster crowed and in the distance a dog was barking. I said, Lord, my Lord, I thank you for your help. Amen, Amen. This concentrated fluid called "Crypto" does wonders.

**Now we understand that Alzheimer's needs:**

Alumina 6x

Arsenicum 6x

Circu-Flow for arterial congestion

Crypto Holy Water from the Chapel of Miracles

**There is a God. He cures. He helps. Amen.**

Rev. Hanna Kroeger
7075 Valmont Road
Boulder, Colorado 80301